SMOOTH

BOOKS BY CELIA BONADUCE

TINY HOUSE NOVELS

Tiny House on the Hill

Tiny House on the Road

Tiny House in the Trees

FAT CHANCE, TEXAS SERIES

Welcome to Fat Chance, Texas

Slim Pickins' in Fat Chance, Texas

Livin' Large in Fat Chance, Texas

VENICE BEACH ROMANCES

The Merchant of Venice Beach

A Comedy of Erinn

Much Ado About Mother

With Jodi Thomas and Rachael Miles

A Texas Kind of Christmas

SMOOTH

life hacks to get you smoothly through chemo

CELIA BONADUCE

Photography & Illustrations by Justine Joy

Published by Geoffrey Spring Books

Book Design, Layout, and Editing by elle fournier/The Paisley Zebra

Print ISBN: 978-1-66789-982-4

eBook ISBN: 978-1-66789-983-1

To Laura—the velvet steamroller.

Thanks for the momentum!

I looked in the mirror

Bald as could be

But then I looked closer

And I was still me

CONTENTS

FOREWORD

Every one of my patients is unique and has a story. And every one of them is truly brave and, in a way, a superhuman. Celia, though, always stood out. It's not that chemotherapy was easy for her or that she didn't have any side effects. But most of the time when I would walk into her room, she still had a wide smile on her face. Believe me, this is not common during full-dose chemotherapy! Her appearance was the same as everyone else. Sometimes she would wear makeup and sometimes not. She never shied away from having a bald head, although sometimes she would sport some fashionable headscarf. But what stood out is that she almost always looked happy.

How was Celia so upbeat through chemotherapy? I don't think this was because she is some Zen master. Part of it was that she had decided she was not going to feel sorry for herself. And the other part was that she used her strength to find ways of making the journey less unpleasant— and they worked! She would tell me about recipes she had discovered, products she had found that soothed her skin, and friends who were supporting her in very concrete ways. The list would go on and on with the ways she had found to make the journey smoother.

I can tell you, they did make a difference.

So I was thrilled when Celia told me she was going to write a book and share what she had found with others. This book is packed with gems of advice. Things that you won't be able to get from your oncologist that make life better while going through chemotherapy. I highly recommend it to every woman going through chemotherapy. You don't have to figure this out all on your own.

Parvin F. Peddi, MD
Division of Hematology & Oncology
University of California, Los Angeles

INTRODUCTION

One test had led to the next and then the next. I'd had two mammograms, an ultrasound, and a biopsy. So when the call came, I was ready.

"Hi, Celia . . ." my doctor said, her voice trailing off. "It's cancer."

"Yeah," I said, picturing my life as a novelist and a TV producer grinding to an immediate halt. "My village would have to be missing its idiot for me to not have suspected this."

So then I did the breast cancer thing—lumpectomy, chemotherapy, and radiation. I learned a lot about breast cancer (for example, that mine was Stage 1-B triple-negative breast cancer). But here's a secret: while there are lots of books out there about women's personal stories during their breast cancer journeys, when you're going through it, you don't give a rat's ass about anyone else's story. You just want to know how to get through it yourself.

This isn't a personal retrospective, nor is it a medical journal. But I do have some recommendations I'd like to pass along—just some ideas that might make your life easier during this most stressful of times. All the products mentioned are my personal favorites from my own chemo adventure. No company has endorsed, sponsored, or bribed me. The photographs of the products are beautiful and professional looking because my beautiful and professional friend Justine shot them.

As you start your journey, you will wonder where you will get the mental as well as physical strength to voluntarily show up for chemo month after month. But you will find that strength or that strength will find you. I hope these tips will make your trip easier.

Because it's all about you.

As it should be.

HAIR LOSS
LIFE HACKS

Discussing hair loss right off the bat might seem like jumping the gun, but let's face it: it's *the* thing that will be on your mind. You might luck out and be the one-in-a-zillion woman who doesn't lose most or all of her hair during chemo. But are you really feeling lucky these days?

The following tips might help.

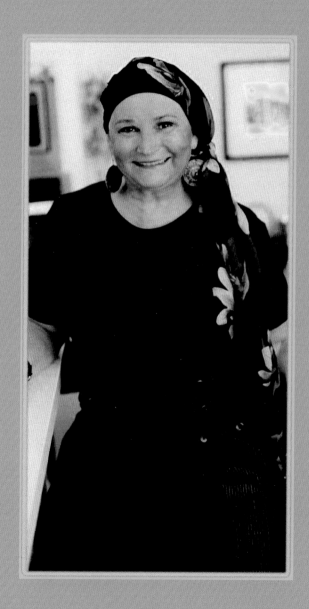

Cutting Your Hair Before Chemo Starts

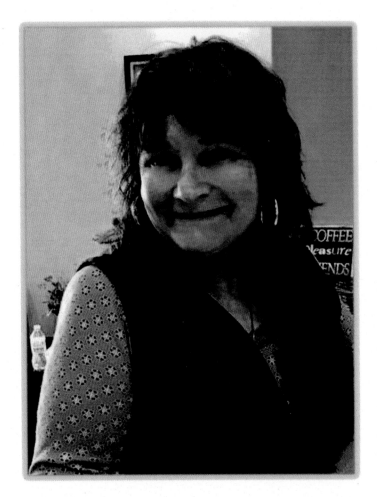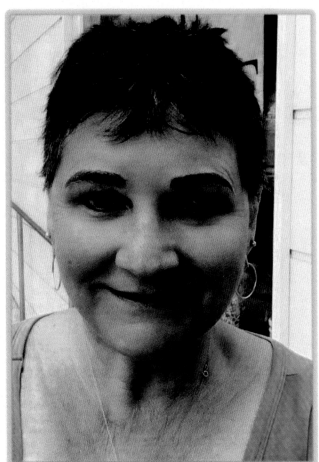

Many women choose to cut their hair short before it starts falling out

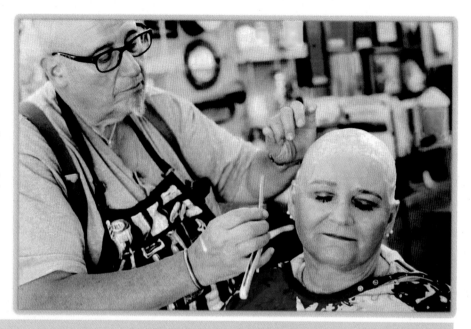

Personal Choice: Limiting the trauma is the name of the game. After one of my friends told me that she decided to try her luck with keeping her hair, then woke up one morning with a fistful of curls on her pillow, I got a pixie cut to limit the emotional damage. This also gave my friends, my family, and me the chance to get used to me with short hair. This worked both as a precursor to baldness and then for the protracted road back to long hair. When my hair started to fall out, I had it straight-razored off at an old-timey barbershop. That experience actually turned out to be kind of fun in the "I have cancer but will focus on everything else" sort of way.

The "Cold Cap"

If you're still on the fence as to whether to cut your hair or hope for the best and not cut it, you'll probably hear about the cold cap—an outer-space-movie-from-the-fifties-looking contraption that sits on your head. Cold caps are no guarantee you won't lose your hair and they aren't recommended for migraine sufferers. They say that after a cold cap regimen, your hair might grow back faster because it doesn't have to grow from below the root. But nobody makes any promises. You might keep most of your hair or some of your hair or none of your hair. Some medical insurance companies don't cover the cost, which can be $400 a session. If the price doesn't scare you away, the cold cap might be something to consider.

Personal Choice: The cold cap did not call to me. I suffer from occasional migraines, had no interest in keeping potentially 50% of my hair, and I'm always cold even without the equivalent of ice cubes on my head.

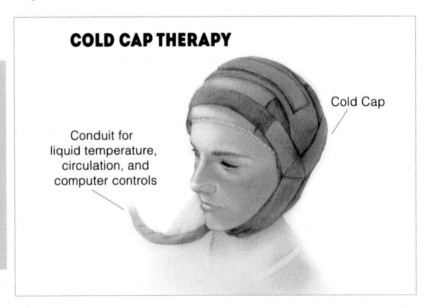

COLD CAP THERAPY

Cold Cap

Conduit for liquid temperature, circulation, and computer controls

Wigs

Chances are good that you'll lose some or all of your hair, so the next reality to face is: what to do about it? Embrace your badass baldness? Get a wig or two or three? Many women take the opportunity to try different textures, colors, and styles. Other women try to duplicate their own hair. It's a good idea to actually go to a store and try on wigs . . . internet shopping can lead to costly and unflattering mistakes, neither of which you need right now. It's worth checking with your insurance company because they might cover the cost.

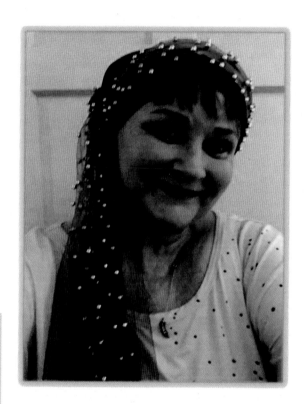

Personal Choice: I was as surprised as anybody that I decided against wigs. Staring at my bald reflection was unnerving enough, but I just felt really alien to myself in hair that wasn't my own. However, I was a huge fan of fake bangs—which, added to scarves and turbans, gave just a hint-o-hair that made me feel a little more confident and healthy looking.

Scarves & Turbans

The internet is awash in gorgeous scarves and turbans. Secondhand stores, fabric stores, and regular old department stores all have wonderful scarves that will spark your imagination. A fabulous diversionary tactic—while not focusing directly on cancer but still feeling proactive—is watching YouTube videos and learning how to tie and wrap scarves.

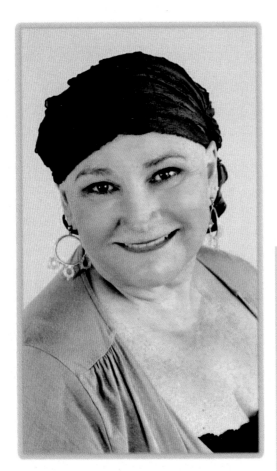

Suburban Turban:

www.suburbanturban.com

Personal Choice: By the time chemo claimed my hair, I had stored up three hatboxes of turbans and scarves. I also bought several pre-tied scarves and turbans, which I thought I'd use in a pinch. Once I was in the thick of it, though, I relied on the pre-tied turbans most of the time. You feel pretty lousy during chemo and tying scarves often seemed like a burden. But having learned some amazing ways to tie scarves, I did employ my new skill to impress my friends.

Scarf Volumizer

The custom of married Orthodox Jewish women to cover their hair led to the popularization of the *tichel*, a head covering that can range from a plain kerchief tied in the back to elaborate wraps and fabrics. Muslim women also cover their hair with a *hijab* for religious reasons. Culture also plays a part in many women's choice of head coverings, including African and Indian women. With all of these women covering their hair, there developed a need for an "undergarment" that created volume. If women with hair needed volume, think how much happier you'll be with a little extra pouf!

Personal Choice: A whole new world opened up as soon as I found this "head underwear." The volumizers come in many shapes, from a modest rounded look to a towering cone. My favorite volumizer comes on a stretchy non-slip headband, with stuffing that can be customized to your scarf-height requirement. And, best of all, they are easy on tender heads.

Wrapunzel:

www.wrapunzel.com

▼ *NO VOLUMIZER*

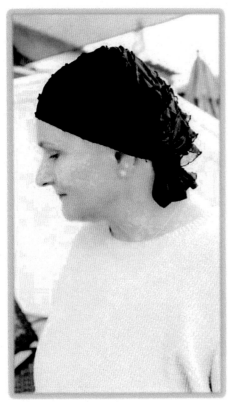

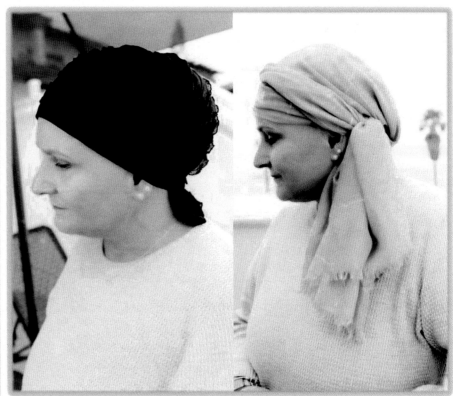

▲ *WITH VOLUMIZER*

8

Donated Scarves, Turbans & Wigs
Are Available to You

If you find yourself in need of some donated wigs or scarves, check out the American Cancer Society. The ACS is one of the best-known cancer awareness organizations with a free wig program. They have local chapters throughout the United States and can guide you to all kinds of support, including donated wigs and scarves. To that end, the American Cancer Society is featured on Headcovers Unlimited's website for a comprehensive, thoughtful online experience.

Cancer Horizons is creating one of the largest directories of FREE hats, scarves, and caps exclusively for cancer patients.

American Cancer Society:	Headcovers Unlimited:	Cancer Horizons:
www.cancer.org	www.headcovers.com	www.cancerhorizons.com

Taking Care of a Bald Head

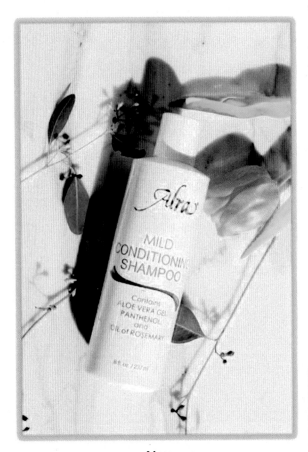

Alra:

www.alra.com

Whether you decide to shave your head voluntarily or just go partially or totally bald from chemotherapy, you will be surprised to find how freaking tender your head becomes. Some people feel pain or itching when their hair falls out. Taking care of your scalp involves as many choices as taking care of your hair. Chemo can make your scalp feel dry or sensitive. The slightest friction can cause irritation, so make sure anything you put on your head—from shampoo to hats—is gentle and non-irritating. Ingredients to look for include soothing aloe vera, pro-vitamin B-5 (called panthenol) for added moisture, and oil of rosemary to help blood circulation.

Personal Choice: I never experienced pain but my head was very tender the entire time I was doing chemo. Alra Mild Conditioning Shampoo, which I also used for a body wash, was extremely soothing.

Eyebrows

While the loss of the hair on your head is the most obvious, be aware that all of the hair on your body is probably going on vacation for the duration of infusions and a few months post-chemo. I was seriously bald as a pear. This includes eyebrows. Most days, you're not going to feel like putting on makeup, but when you do, have a plan for those brows . . . because you're going to have to guess where they were.

Personal Choice: Microblading is a fancy way of saying "eyebrow tattoos with feathery strokes." Knowing I was going to be losing my brows, I opted to tattoo some brows before chemo struck. This was one of the best things I did for myself. I've already had tattooed eyeliner for years, so this wasn't too much of a stretch. I highly recommend doing both. It really did help me think I looked better than I felt.

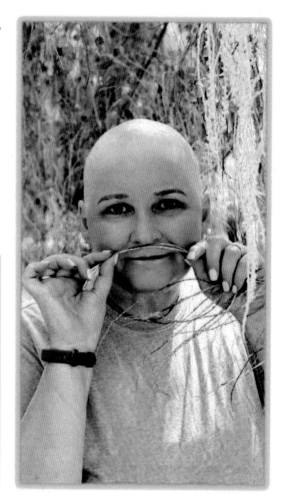

Eyelashes

Yes, eyelashes go too.

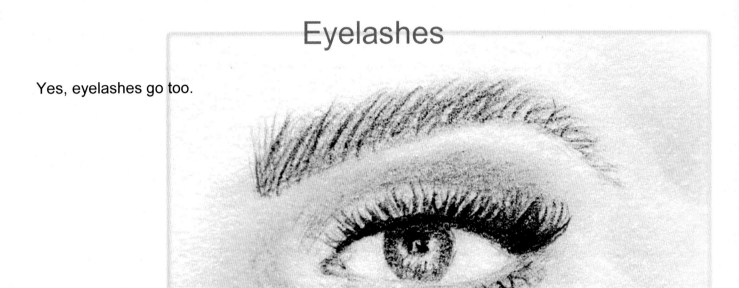

Personal Choice: I thought I would outfox the eyelash thieves and used one of those eyelash lengtheners you brush on every day. Two things went wrong: One, I really didn't feel like brushing my teeth, let alone applying an eyelash lengthener every day. And two, my tear ducts clogged, giving me a pink stye (because the Chemo Gods apparently do not take kindly to intervention). On days when I was feeling pretty well (and there were many of those days in the third week after chemo), I conjured up a skill that had lain dormant since high school: I applied false eyelashes. Apparently, it's like riding a bicycle. You never forget how to do it.

SKIN, NAILS & MOUTH
LIFE HACKS

Chemo does a real number on your skin. Itchiness, rashes, dryness, tenderness, and sun sensitivity will vie to outdo each other during treatment. Luckily, there are enough prescription and over-the-counter creams and drugs to keep the worst at bay.

The following tips might help.

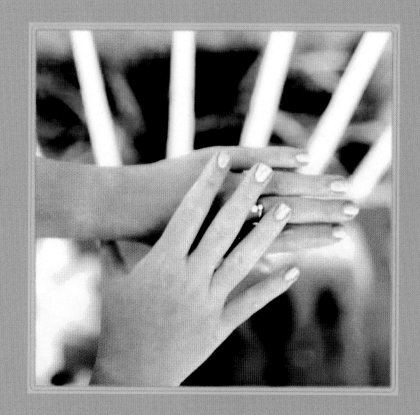

Skin Care

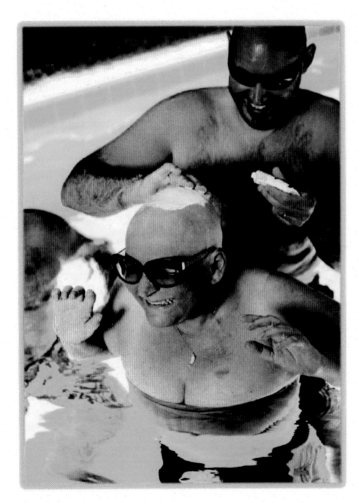

Itching is a very common side effect of chemo. Different chemo medications cause different reasons for itching and you'll need a professional to guide you. Don't try to tough this one out. Call your nurse or doctor immediately.

Once you're past the diagnosis stage and you are left with your official treatment regime, do not forget good skin care, which will help reduce itching. Maintaining a cool room temperature, using gentle soaps, shampoos, and laundry soaps, and frequent use of fragrance-free lotions will all help.

Sunscreen

Oncologists will be very clear: Chemotherapy can often make patients more sensitive to the sun. The sun's rays are strongest between 10:00 a.m. and 3:00 p.m., so limiting your exposure during those hours is a good idea. Always use sunscreen with an SPF of 30 or higher and reapply it throughout the day if you're going to be outside for any length of time.

Supergoop! Sunscreen:

www.supergoop.com

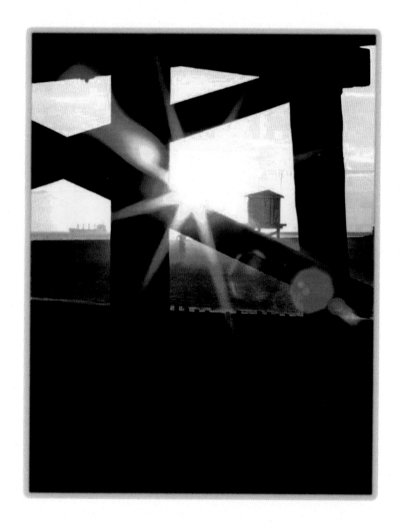

Arm Sleeves

Even if you've never had sensitive skin, chemo might change all that. Some of chemo's all-too-common side effects include dry skin, flushing (a temporary redness of the face and/or neck caused by dilation of the blood capillaries), hyperpigmentation (darkening of the skin, which can be an overall or localized darkening), and—my personal bugaboo—chemo rash.

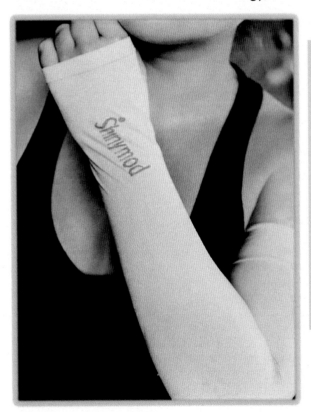

Personal Choice: On my good days, I would relish getting out for a drive. I felt happy to be connected to the world without straining my limited energy. While the Southern California sun can be a pleasure, it can be too much of a good thing during chemo. Sunscreen was never enough to protect my hands and arms from the sun when I was driving. My husband found these arm sleeves for me. They cover your arms from fingertips to biceps—and the freedom from the sun they afford is epic!

Shinymod Arm Sleeves:

www.shinymod.com

Aveeno Products

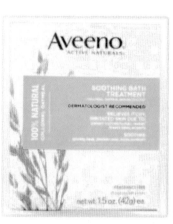

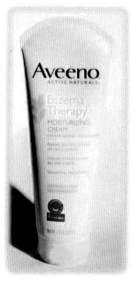

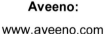

Aveeno:

www.aveeno.com

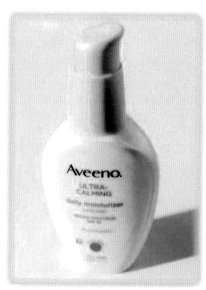

Personal Choices: Warm (not hot) baths and the use of Aveeno's Soothing Bath Treatment with colloidal oatmeal got me through many an itch-fest. I was also at war with dry skin and I combatted that by slathering myself in Aveeno's Eczema Therapy Moisturizing Cream.

Aveeno Ultra-Calming Daily Moisturizer is perfect for soothing irritated, dry skin without feeling overly heavy. The information on the box says that the formula features calming feverfew and nourishing oat, two of nature's most effective and clinically-proven ingredients for sensitive skin. While I'll have to take their word for it, I can tell you from personal experience, it works.

Skin Scrub

Chemo can cause your skin to have one or more reactions, none of them good. Your skin can become dry, itchy, flaky, swollen, or puffy. Or you may develop sores that become painful, wet, and infected. Bottom line: your skin will be very sensitive and your usual skincare regimen will probably have to be rethought.

Personal Choice: I have always been a fan of exfoliating with walnut scrubs, but found them too harsh for my new delicate chemo skin. I discovered SUGAR scrubs were perfect. Scooping out a little delicately scented scrub, I could control the roughness of the exfoliation by holding my hand under the showerhead until the sugar was a consistency my skin could tolerate. The internet is full of recipes for making your own sugar scrubs and I salute you if you feel like making an exfoliant while going through chemo. Personally, I found Tree Hut Shea Sugar Scrub in Tropical Mango to be just lovely.

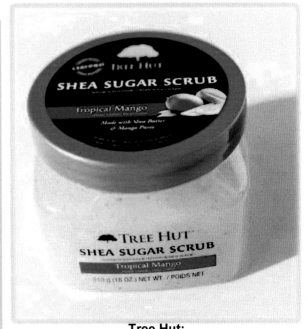

Tree Hut:

www.treehutshea.com

18

Mouth & Teeth

Chemo can play havoc with your mouth. When your oncologist recommends a visit to the dentist to make sure your teeth, gums, and mouth are in good shape before you start treatment, listen to her. While adding a trip to the dentist is probably the very last thing you want to do, chemo has been known to affect the entire mouth, so you 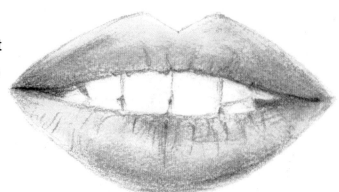 want to make sure your teeth and gums are in good condition at the outset. Two common side effects of chemo are severe dry mouth and blistering inside your mouth. It's called "chemo mouth" and it's nothing to smirk at! Tell your dentist that you're about to embark on a chemo adventure. He or she will probably recommend a mouthwash with no alcohol or sugar. You can also rinse with a homemade mouthwash made with one quart of water and one teaspoon of baking soda.

Personal Choice: I struggled with mouth sores and found relief in a very odd place—my keep-my-teeth-from-grinding night guard. The dental guard kept the inside of my cheeks off my teeth, which created a barrier between the tooth enamel and the sores. I used the night guard religiously during treatment (which, don't tell my dentist, was not the case before chemo)—not only at night but anytime the mouth sores were bothering me.

Dry Mouth

Dry mouth sounds so benign—until you experience it. It should be called SAHARA DESERT MOUTH. As in, stick-to-the-roof-of-your-mouth dry. This is caused by chemotherapy making the saliva thicker. Radiation will also mess with your salivary glands. In any case, this unpleasant side effect usually clears up within two weeks to two **months** of your chemo/radiation graduation.

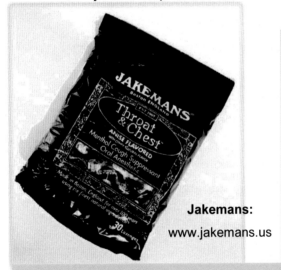

Jakemans:
www.jakemans.us

Personal Choices:

Dry mouth was a huge issue for me both day and night. Most of the cough drops I tried only helped with the dryness while I was sucking on them. I was looking for a low-sugar or sugar-free cough drop with natural ingredients that included a soothing oil. I found Jakeman's Throat & Chest Drops. These little guys will be your new best friends. They keep your mouth moist long after the last sliver has dissolved.

Dry mouth also causes chapped or split lips. I probably bought every lip balm on the market—not that I was ever dissatisfied with any of them, but I was always finding myself without one. (I'm still finding them in my pockets, purses, suitcases, and backpacks.) One very gentle lip balm favorite was by L'Occitane.

L'Occitane:
www.loccitane.com

Nails

In case you forgot learning this in high school biology, hair and nails are basically made up of the same protein: keratin. Because chemo drugs are hell-bent on rapidly dividing hair follicle cells, your nails will probably not be spared. Fingernails and toenails often become weak during chemo, causing them to separate and sometimes fall off. Unfortunately, there is no way to completely avoid this. Basically, just one more thing that sucks about chemo.

Nails have always been a big deal to me, so when my oncologist told me that my nails would not support acrylics or gel manicures, I cried like she was going to weigh me in public. Fingernails and toenails are compromised during chemo, becoming weak and brittle. Lots of really unattractive things can happen—Beau's lines (horizontal or vertical lines that appear darker or lighter than the rest of your nail), yellow nails, or total loss of your nails. Fingernail loss is more common than toenail loss. Sometimes, fingernails can come off long after treatment.

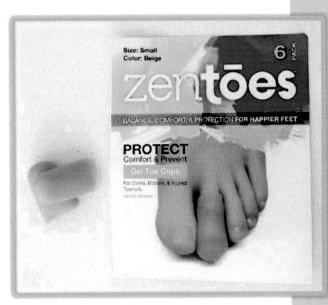

Zentoes:

www.zentoes.com

Personal Choice: I followed my doctor's orders and took off my acrylic nails. I did my research, switched to a breathable nail polish, and thought I was home free. But I still had problems. Several of my fingernails came off months after chemo ended. The worst part of having no fingernails was how sensitive my skin became. Typing, opening a pop-top can, and texting were exercises in masochism. I randomly came across a godsend called Zentoes, a gel cap that protects the toes from blisters, corns, and toe pain (while also moisturizing the skin). I stuck them on my missing fingernails and, while they are never going to be the next fashion trend, they made life bearable.

MAKEUP
LIFE HACKS

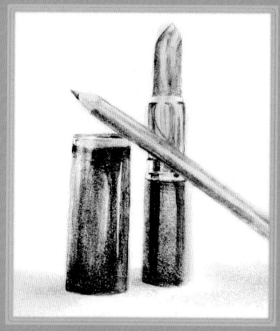

The harsh reality is: makeup will probably not be a priority during the dog days of chemo. But on your good days, you might just feel like dusting yourself off and looking as spectacular as possible. Putting on a pretty dress, your best wig or eye-catching scarf, earrings, and a little makeup can do wonders for the soul and make you feel like you're giving the middle finger to chemo. The key words here are "a little" makeup—now is not the time to mask your sensitive skin with layers of heavy foundation and powder blush.

I've always loved makeup, so investigating what products would be best for my chemo journey was not exactly a hardship. I've also always used a moisturizer and gone for a natural look, so I didn't have to kick my whole look to the curb once my skin became sensitive. The good news is: I loved the look these products gave me, and continue to use them months after chemo ended and my skin regained its normal texture.

Lips

Chemo treatments that affect the inside of your mouth will also dry out your lips—which can result in dry, cracked skin. Anyone who has survived a blustery day (remember when mere chapped lips felt like a tragedy?) knows that chapped lips are susceptible to bleeding and blistering. It's like that. Only more so.

Originally, I used a tinted lip balm as my lipstick, but I kept forgetting it was tinted and would slather it on like a transparent lip balm. I would get weird glances everywhere I went until I caught sight of myself in a mirror. The colored balm, applied erratically an inch or so above and below my lips, made me look like I was headed to clown school. So, first up: lip balm is lip balm and lipstick is lipstick.

Personal Choice: The absolute best moisturizing lipstick I found is made by City Lips. I almost didn't try City Lips because they advertise themselves as a "plumping" lip gloss. I found that plumping lipsticks and glosses tend to make your lips "tingle" (an advertising word for "stings"), which hurt just thinking about it. But City Lips also used words that hit home, like "moisturizing" and "long-term solution" and "deep hydration." Add a zillion pretty colors and I was a goner.

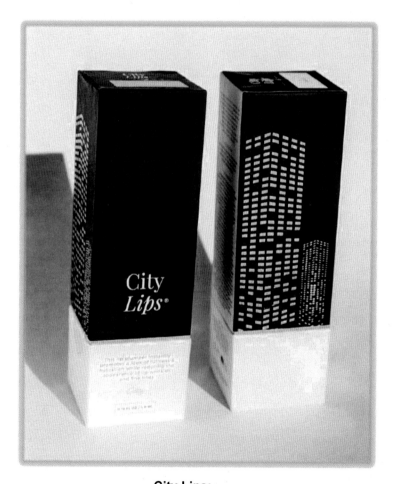

City Lips:

www.citybeauty.com

Eyes

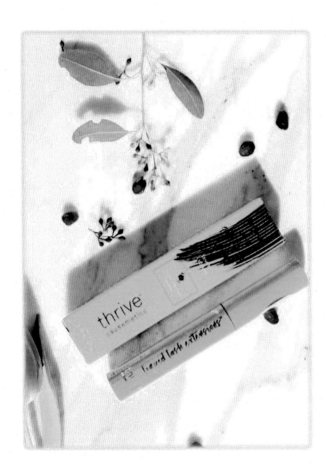

Accept the fact that you will not be able to outwit chemo drugs. If they want anything remotely connected to hair follicles, they will lay waste to not only your hair and nails but also to your eyelashes. Same drugs, different cosmetic misfortune.

Personal Choice: My eyelashes didn't entirely disappear until pretty late in the game, so I made the most of what I had with mascara by Thrive Causemetics. Thrive has great products but an even greater story behind it. Thrive was created by makeup artist Karissa Bodnar who lost her 24-year-old friend Kristy to cancer. Karissa established Thrive Causemetics in Kristy's honor. Thrive also donates a portion of their profits to empowering women. The mascara is fantastically lush and non-irritating, checking off the final box of "why to use Thrive."

Thrive Causemetics:

www.thrivecausemetics.com

Boom! Products

Personal Choice: I also started using Boom Cosmetics by Cindy Joseph. Cindy calls her three-pack of products "Color," "Glo," and "Glimmer" and they're advertised as "Your entire makeup bag in three sticks." Sounded good to me! The boomsticks can be used as blush, lipstick, eye shadow, highlighter, moisturizer, and more. The result is healthy, natural-looking skin, which seemed an impossibility at the time I ordered it. In the middle of my own journey, Cindy, the creator of Boom Cosmetics, died from cancer. I felt I had lost a friend.

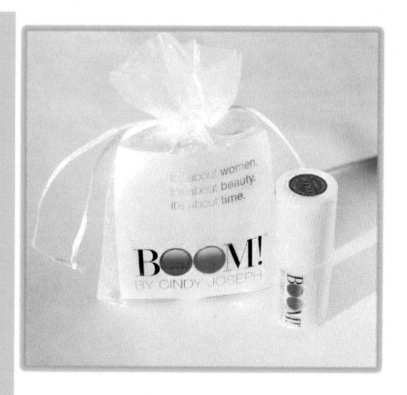

Boom! Cosmetics by Cindy Joseph:
www.boombycindyjoseph.com

CLOTHES
LIFE HACKS

In general, one of the most common side effects of chemotherapy is fatigue. Napping and resting will become part of your daily routine, so comfort will be the name of the game. Cotton, brushed cotton, flannel, cashmere, and cashmere/cotton blends all feel incredibly good on delicate skin. Beware of elastic touching your skin and make sure waistbands and bras don't pinch. These can be uncomfortable when you are trying to sleep and can also cause welts. Chemo also increases the risk of vaginal infections, so cotton underwear is essential.

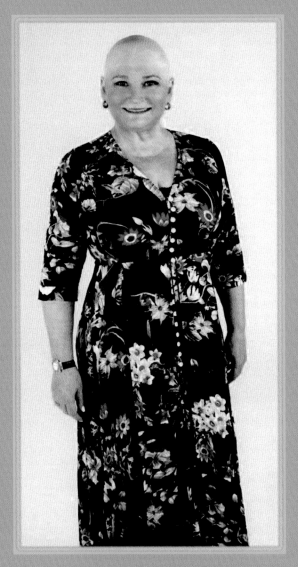

Dressing for Ports

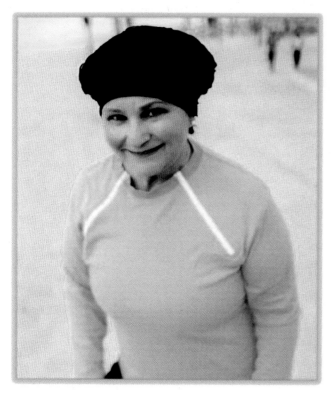

Some patients may have the option of getting their chemotherapy infusion through their veins or via a port. It was recommended that I opt for the port, so I did. A small disc about the size of a quarter was inserted into my chest during a short outpatient surgery a few days before I started chemo. It's placed under the skin and mine was, according to my nurses, beautifully placed and barely visible. But maybe they say that to all the girls. In any case, a thin, flexible tube connects the port to a large vein in the chest. Chemotherapy medicines flow through a special needle that fits right into the port. It makes the needle virtually painless. Chest ports require some extra consideration: On infusion days, it's helpful for you and your chemo nurse if you're wearing an easily accessible top.

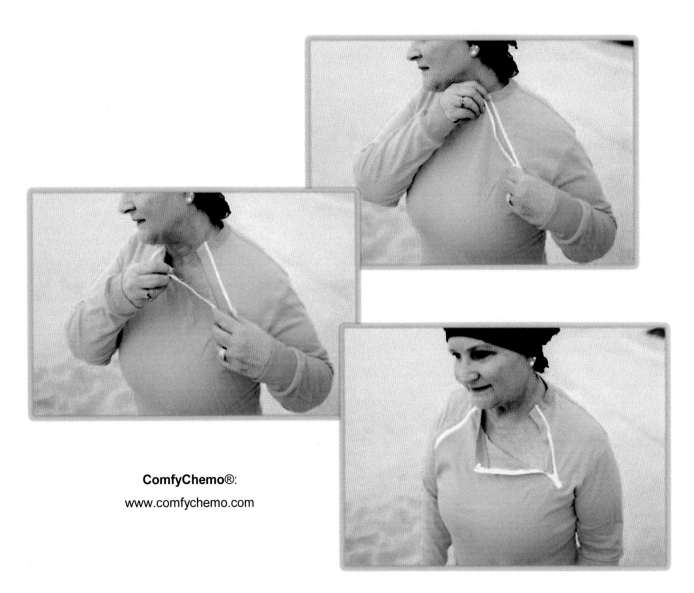

ComfyChemo®:

www.comfychemo.com

30

Being Comfy

You know the expression "Clothes make the man?" I took that to heart during chemo, but altered it. My mantra was "Pajamas make the woman." I'm a huge eBay shopper and bought flannel PJ bottoms in cute colors and patterns for a few dollars each. On non-chemo days, I paired these with coordinating T-shirts from Gildan. I always ironed the pajama bottoms, so it appeared I was going for this look on purpose. When I had a scheduled infusion, I would swap the T-shirt for one of the three (green, pink, and black) chemo-specific shirts I bought from ComfyChemo®. These creative inventions are made from a heavy T-shirt material with two zippers at the neckline, which can be unzipped to expose the port while leaving the rest of your chest covered and saving your real shirts from being stretched out at the neck. The shirts are beautifully made and designed. With my bald head and crew neck ComfyChemo® shirt, I looked like a Starship commander (in pajama bottoms).

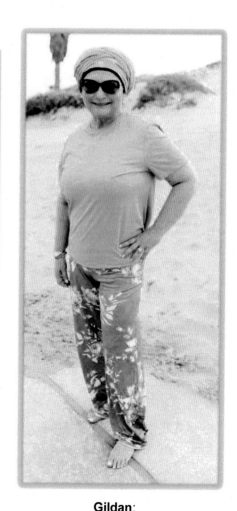

Gildan:

www.gildan.com

Comfy Outfit Combos

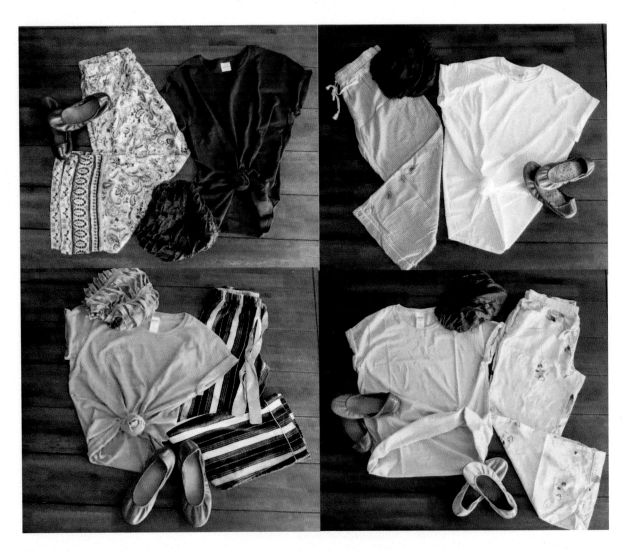

Bras

Bra research was naturally a roller-coaster ride. I had a lumpectomy that made my affected boob slightly smaller than it was initially and obviously also smaller than the unaffected boob. The difference was noticeable in structured bras. I also wanted a cotton, non-binding, non-underwire bra. Basically, I needed a supportive bra that wouldn't poke, chafe, or irritate me. I had just about given up when I found a cotton, non-underwire, wide strap, seven-hook, front closure bra called "The Meryl" by Leading Lady. It was so cozy, I could sleep in it. If it ever felt uncomfortable, all I had to do was unfasten one or two of the bottom hooks. These are still my go-to bras.

Leading Lady:

www.leadinglady.com

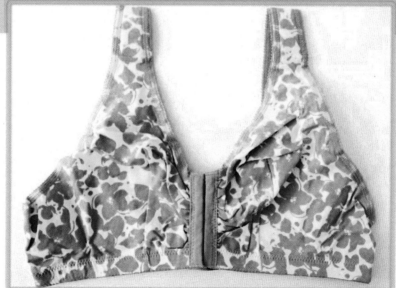

THINGS PEOPLE SAY

Your skin isn't the only thing that will
be hypersensitive during chemo.
People will say things that will really,
really bug you.

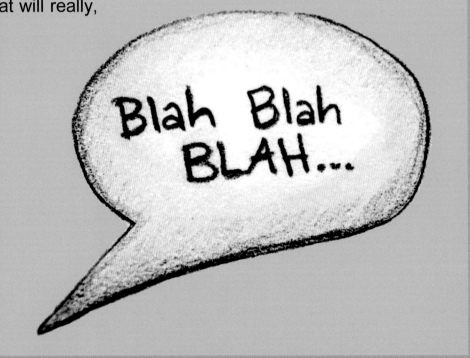

People Will Say Things Like . . .

- "I always wanted to shave my head."

- "My aunt had breast cancer—and she died." (*person starts crying*)

- "I'm afraid you're going to die." (*person starts crying*)

- "You got this!" (*there are days when this is completely fine, but there are days when you don't feel like "you got this" and you think you're letting everybody down*)

- "I don't believe in western medicine."

- "My sister didn't miss a day of work."

I realized that everyone was just as freaked out by my cancer and by my appearance as I was and just didn't know what to say.

I chose to hear "I love you" no matter what was being said.

It's also not a bad idea to have a list of things to offer should someone say, "If there is anything I can do, let me know." You probably already know which of your friends are just paying lip service and which friends truly want to help.

Don't Be Shy

Almost everyone will say, "If there is anything I can do, let me know." And, while they may not come up with anything to do on their own, most people will be thrilled to lend a hand when you need it. And you will need help—rides to chemo, shopping, a quick run to the pharmacy, the list goes on. Some can be organized ahead of time, but many things pop up out of the blue.

You will be surprised how many of your friends and family will step up IF YOU ASK.

Here Are Things I Asked For—and Got!

♥ Nourishing comfort food. I knew my mother was going to make batches of homemade soups for me. We were planning to follow *The Cancer-Fighting Kitchen* cookbook by Rebecca Katz and I asked my vegan niece Countess to make me twelve quarts of *The Cancer-Fighting Kitchen*'s vegan broth, which she froze in quart-size containers. My friend Laura did the same with the cookbook's bone broth. My mom would wake me up with a homemade soup every day. There is no denying that eating well—and right—will make a huge difference in how you feel.

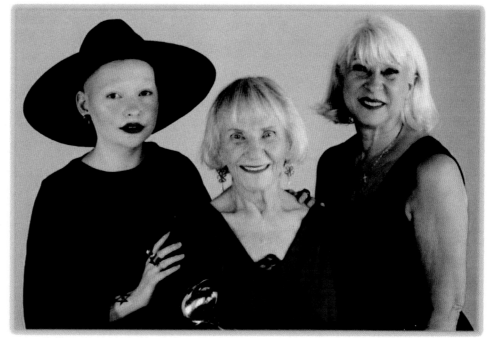

TEAM SOUP:
Countess, Mom & Laura

♥ Texts, not phone calls. Chemo leaves you exhausted. Friends and family mean well, but there are days when you'll be just too tired to talk. If everyone checks in by text, you can decide when and if you have enough energy to return the text—or, if you're feeling perky (and there are days when you probably will), you can call.

♥ Help with my book. My friends Laura and Justine worked for months on this book!

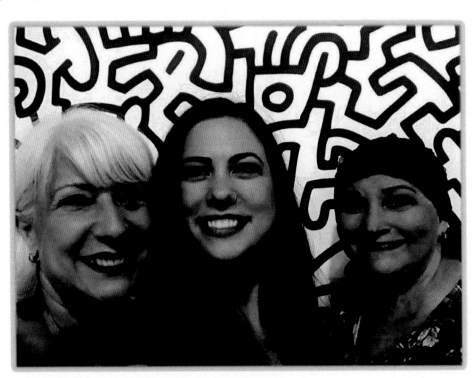

Things I Didn't Ask For—and Got!

♥ Friends understanding when I either canceled or bailed early.

♥ My mother's love and unswerving attention throughout my journey. She was my "day care"—in her 300-ft. tiny house. One day, when I was returning to my place on her couch from a trip to the bathroom, my mom said, "Hello there, pretty little bald head." Now that's love.

♥ Husband, friends, and family never making me feel like an imposition.

♥ Snail mail cards and postcards—declarations of love that I could read on my own time.

♥ Letters that I could hold in my hand, which seemed so permanent and made cancer seem more fleeting. The cancer would be gone but my letters would still be with me.

My niece and namesake, Celia, Jr., was in medical school at the time that I was diagnosed. She said that watching me deal with cancer has made her a better doctor. She saw up close that you had to see the person as well as the disease. I will forever treasure her letter.

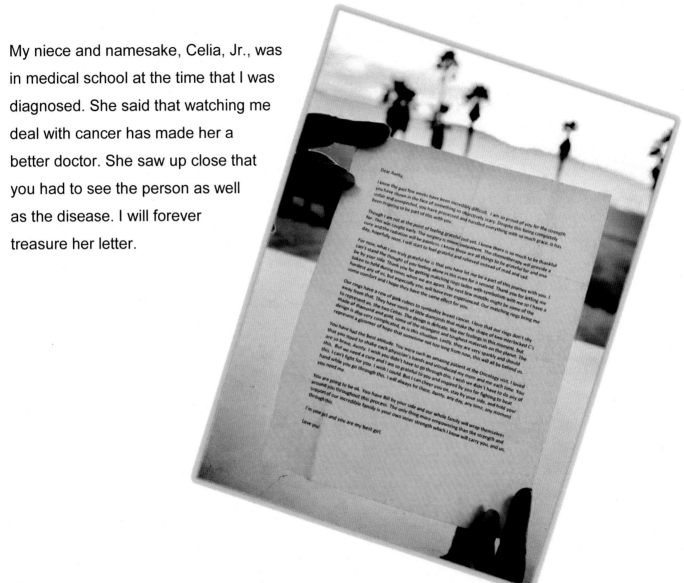

Dear Aunty,

I know the past few weeks have been incredibly difficult. I am so proud of you for the strength you have shown in the face of something so objectively scary. Despite this being completely unfair and unexpected, you have processed and handled everything with so much grace. It has been inspiring to be a part of this with you.

Though I am not at the point of feeling grateful just yet, I know there is so much to be thankful for. This was caught early. The surgery is minor/outpatient. The chemotherapy will provide a cure and the radiation will be painless. I know these are all things to be grateful for and one day, hopefully soon, I will start to feel grateful and relieved instead of mad and sad.

For now, what I am truly grateful for is that you have let me be a part of this journey with you. I can't stand the thought of you feeling alone in this even for a second. Thank you for letting me be by your side. Thank you for getting matching rings laden with symbolism with me so I have a token to hold during times when we are apart. The next few months might be some of the hardest any of us, but especially you, will have ever experienced. Our matching rings bring me some comfort and I hope they have the same effect for you.

Our rings have a row of pink rubies to symbolize breast cancer. I love that our rings don't shy away from that. They have swirls of little diamonds that make the shape of two interlocked C's to represent us, the two Celias. The design is delicate, like our feelings in this moment, but made of diamond and gold, some of the strongest and toughest materials on the planet. The design is also very complicated, as is this situation. Lastly, they are very sparkly and should represent a glimmer of hope that sometime not too long from now, this will all be behind us.

You have had the best attitude. You were such an amazing patient at the Oncology visit. I loved that you stood to shake each physician's hands and introduced my mom and me each time. You are so brave, Aunty. I wish you didn't have to go through this. I wish we didn't have to do any of this. But we need a cure and I am so grateful to you and inspired by you for fighting to beat this. I can't fight for you. I wish I could. But I can cheer you on, stay by your side, and hold your hand while you go through this. I will always be there, Aunty, any day, any time, any moment you need me.

You are going to be ok. You have Bill by your side and our whole family will wrap themselves around you throughout this process. The only thing more empowering than the strength and support of our incredible family is your own inner strength which I know will carry you, and us, through this.

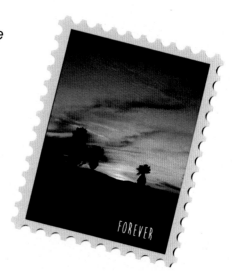

I'm your girl and you are my best girl.

Love you!

Cancer reverberates not only through your healthy cells but psychologically through your friends and family, as well. Don't focus on the people who absent themselves from your journey. They're just scared and their own guilt will be your reward when you're on the other side (smiley face implied). Instead, bask in the love of those who rally.

My niece sent me this letter early in the game. The rings she speaks about were her idea. We went shopping for matching rings so that not only could I take her with me through infusions, she could keep me with her as she finished medical school. I will always cherish her idea, her love, and her letter.

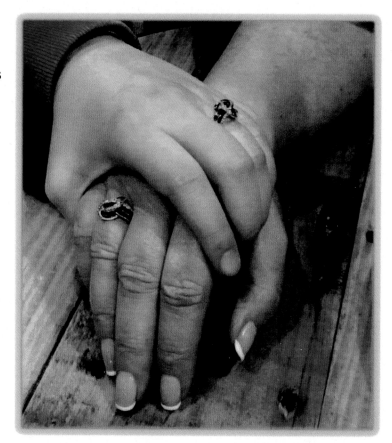

FOOD & RECIPES

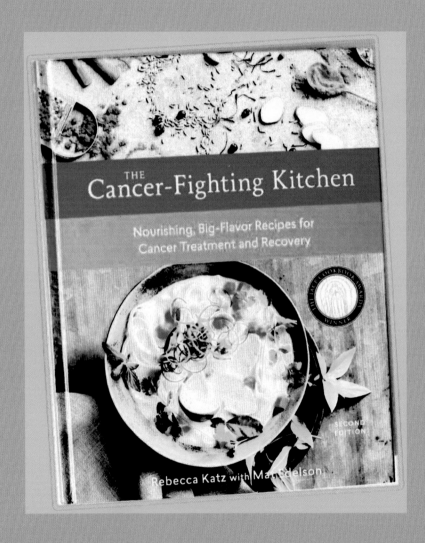

THE
Cancer-Fighting Kitchen

Nourishing, Big-Flavor Recipes for
Cancer Treatment and Recovery

SECOND
EDITION

Rebecca Katz with Mat Edelson

Eating During Chemo

There is so much advice about eating during chemo, it will make your bald head spin. One constant: your taste buds will not be constant! The best advice I got was from my UCLA chemotherapy oncologist, Dr. Parvin Peddi, who did not mince words:

"If you want to eat it, eat it. But don't stock up, because your tastebuds could change tomorrow."

Along with your fickle taste buds, you'll also need to take into account the almost gothic assortment of symptoms from chemo—everything from anemia to bowel ailments to low white blood cell counts.

Eating can be a roller-coaster ride.

Personal Choice: I recommend the cookbook *THE CANCER-FIGHTING KITCHEN* by Rebecca Katz. Not only does it contain over 200 pages of amazing recipes, there's also a list of what to eat for whatever is currently ailing you. I've bought this book for everyone I know who has told me, "I've been diagnosed with cancer." And several of the recipes have become staples in my new healthful life. The recipes sometimes include head-scratching ingredients like *kombu* or *juniper berries*, but there is no need to race all over town searching for them—Amazon has what you need!

Magic Mineral Broth
(The Rosetta Stone of Soup)

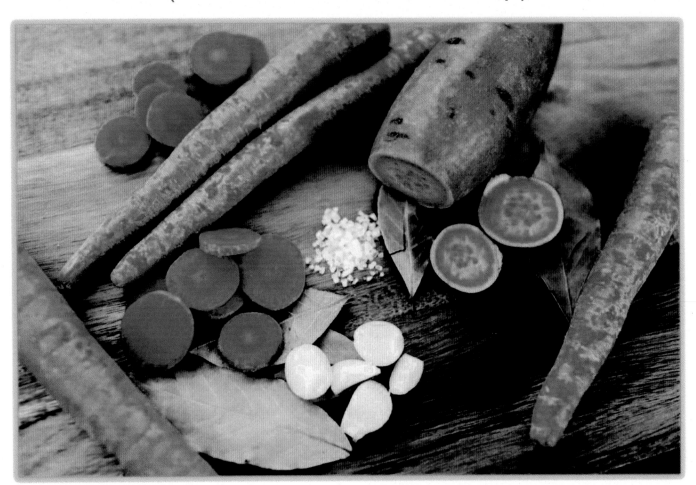

INGREDIENTS:

(Makes 6 quarts)

6 unpeeled carrots, cut into thirds

2 unpeeled yellow onions, cut into chunks

1 leek, white and green parts, cut into thirds

1 bunch celery, including the heart, cut into thirds

4 unpeeled red potatoes, quartered

2 unpeeled Japanese or regular sweet potatoes, quartered

1 unpeeled Garnet sweet potato, quartered

5 unpeeled garlic cloves, halved

½ bunch fresh flat-leaf parsley

1 (8-inch) strip of kombu

12 black peppercorns

4 whole allspice or juniper berries

2 bay leaves

8 quarts cold, filtered water

1 teaspoon sea salt

DIRECTIONS:

Rinse all vegetables well, including the kombu. In a 12-quart or larger stockpot, combine the carrots, onions, leek, celery, red potatoes, sweet potatoes, garlic, parsley, kombu, peppercorns, allspice berries, and bay leaves. Fill the pot with the water to 2 inches below the rim, cover and bring to a boil.

Remove the lid, decrease the heat to low, and simmer, uncovered, for at least 2 hours. As the broth simmers, some of the water will evaporate; add more if the vegetables begin to peek out. Simmer until the full richness of the vegetables can be tasted.

Strain the broth through a large, course-mesh sieve (remember to use a heat-resistant container underneath), then add salt to taste. Let cool to room temperature before refrigerating or freezing.

Cook's Notes:

Like fine wine, this broth gets better with age. The longer the simmer time, the better-tasting and more nutrient-dense the broth will be.

Kombu is dark brown seaweed (kelp) that is dried and folded into sheets. It's used in Japanese cooking to add depth and flavor to soups and stocks. It also adds a tremendous amount of valuable trace minerals to this broth. Look for it in the Asian section of many groceries stores or find it online.

Minestrone

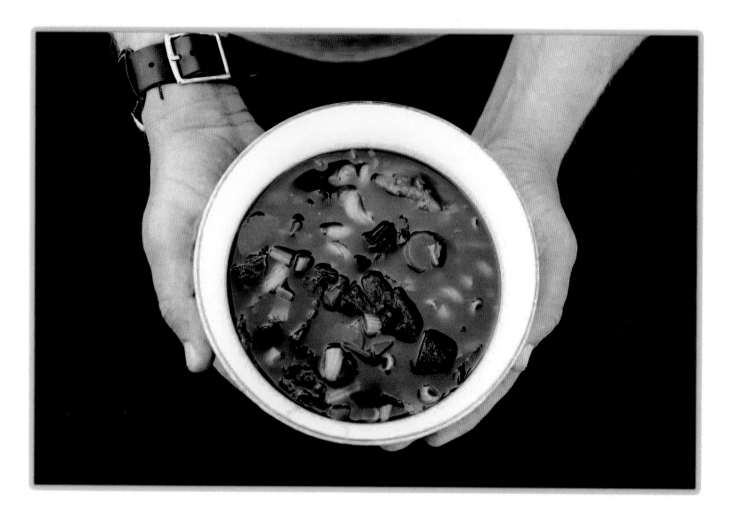

INGREDIENTS:

2 tablespoons extra-virgin olive oil

1 cup finely diced yellow onion

Sea salt

1 cup peeled and finely diced carrot

1 cup finely diced celery

1 cup finely diced zucchini

½ teaspoon finely chopped garlic

½ teaspoon dried oregano

¼ teaspoon dried thyme

¼ teaspoon fennel seeds, crushed

Pinch of red pepper flakes

8 cups Magic Mineral Broth, Chicken Magic Mineral Broth (recipe also in cookbook), or store-bought organic stock

1 (14-oz) can crushed tomatoes

2 cups cooked red kidney beans, or 1 (15-oz) can, rinsed, drained, and mixed with a spritz of fresh lemon juice and a pinch of salt

2 cups stemmed and finely chopped Swiss chard

4 ounces whole grain pasta, cooked

¼ cup finely chopped fresh parsley

Grated organic Parmesan cheese, for garnish (optional)

DIRECTIONS:

Heat the olive oil in a soup pot over medium heat, then add the onion and a pinch of salt and sauté until golden, about 5 minutes. Add the carrot, celery, zucchini, garlic, oregano, thyme, fennel, red pepper flakes, and ¼ teaspoon of salt and sauté for about 4 minutes. Pour in ½ cup of the broth to deglaze the pot and cook until the liquid is reduced by half.

Add the remaining 7½ cups broth, the tomatoes, and the beans and bring to a boil, then lower the heat and simmer for 20 minutes.

Stir in the chard and another ¼ teaspoon salt and cook for 3 minutes more. Stir in the pasta and the parsley. Serve with a sprinkling of Parmesan, if desired.

Curry Cauliflower Soup

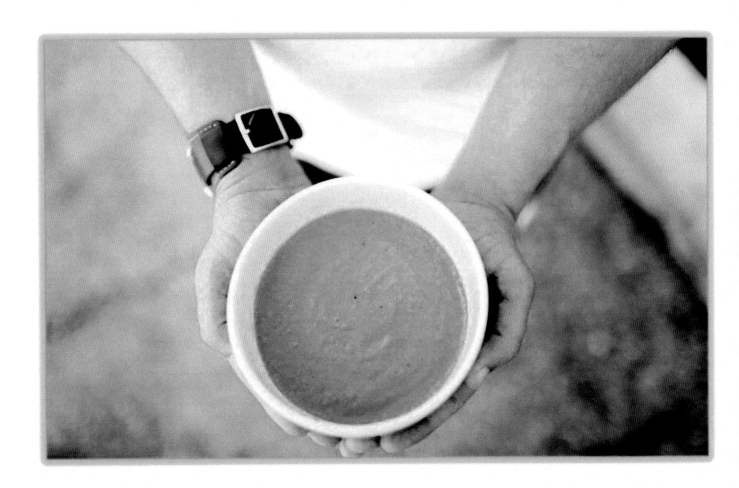

INGREDIENTS:

1 head cauliflower, cut into florets

3 tablespoons extra-virgin olive oil

Sea salt

1 cup finely diced yellow onion

2 carrots, peeled and diced small

1 cup finely diced celery

2 teaspoons curry powder

½ teaspoon ground cumin

½ teaspoon ground coriander

¼ teaspoon ground cinnamon

6 cups Magic Mineral Broth

½ teaspoon lemon juice (optional)

DIRECTIONS:

Preheat oven to 400°F and line a baking sheet with parchment paper.

Toss the cauliflower with 1 tablespoon of the olive oil and ¼ teaspoon of salt, then spread it in an even layer on the prepared pan. Bake until the cauliflower is tender, about 25 minutes.

While the cauliflower is roasting, heat the remaining 2 tablespoons olive oil in a sauté pan over medium heat, then add the onion and a pinch of salt and sauté until translucent, about 3 minutes. Add the carrots, celery, and ¼ teaspoon salt and sauté until the vegetables begin to brown, about 12 minutes.

Add the curry powder, cumin, coriander, cinnamon, and another ½ teaspoon of salt and stir until the spices have coated the vegetables. Pour in ½ cup of broth to deglaze the pan and cook until the liquid is reduced by half. Remove from the heat.

Pour 3 cups of the remaining broth into a blender, then add half of the sautéed vegetables and roasted cauliflower. Blend until smooth, then pour the mixture into a soup pot and repeat the process with the remaining 2½ cups broth and the remaining vegetables and cauliflower. (For a thinner consistency, use another cup of broth.)

Gently reheat the soup over low heat, then taste. You may want to add a spritz of fresh lemon juice and another ¼ teaspoon salt.

BEYOND THE PAIL

There is no denying, no matter how upbeat your doctors are about your prognosis, that a diagnosis of breast cancer can't help but leave you staring mortality in the face. That feeling of "I'm invincible" just seems like the cosmos shaking its head and smirking at you. Don't fight it. You'll be wasting your time on a "Bucket List" just to prove the cosmos wrong. Trust me, you're going to be too tired to go to China.

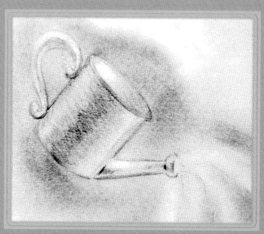

But it's important to keep your mind—and your body—as active as your rounds of chemo will allow. Because a bucket list proved too strenuous, I came up with what I called "Beyond the Pail" . . . a teeny bucket list. Instead of China, I decided I should go into a crazy little run-down but interesting-looking store I'd been passing for 30 years. The fact that the store wasn't worth the trip was beside the point. I had the time, I had the inclination, I did it. Take that, cosmos.

Exercise

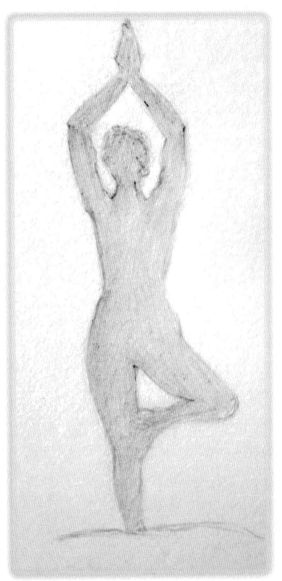

Chemo is a bitch. The whole game is to make it YOUR bitch. It's important to keep the medicine moving through your system. That means exercise, whether you like it or not. Gentle exercise like walking, Pilates, or yoga comes highly recommended if your treatment allows.

Personal Choice: My doctor told me that it was important for the first two days after the infusion (when I felt pretty good anyway) to walk. Although I found it hard to comply as treatment wore on and I wore out, I always did this. I could see the difference in my energy level versus the lethargy in some of my chemo neighbors, who confessed to staying in bed watching TV.

I Danced

Before my diagnosis, I was taking a Pilates class and was pleasantly surprised that I could (sporadically) continue with it. I started taking private lessons instead of classes, as a precaution that I wouldn't overdo it in order to prove that I was Superwoman (it happens). I also managed a private dance lesson or two. In all honesty, while I was not capable of expending a whole lot of energy, there is nothing like getting dressed up and dancing to make you feel like you are still part of life.

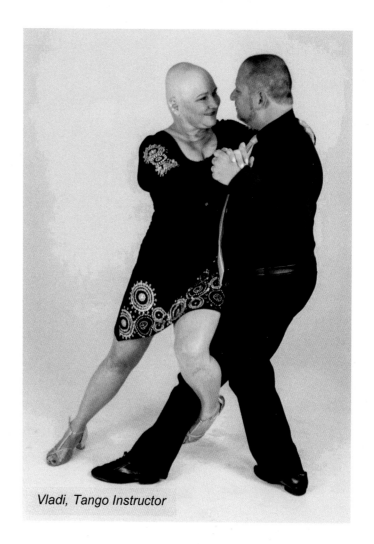

Vladi, Tango Instructor

Chin Up

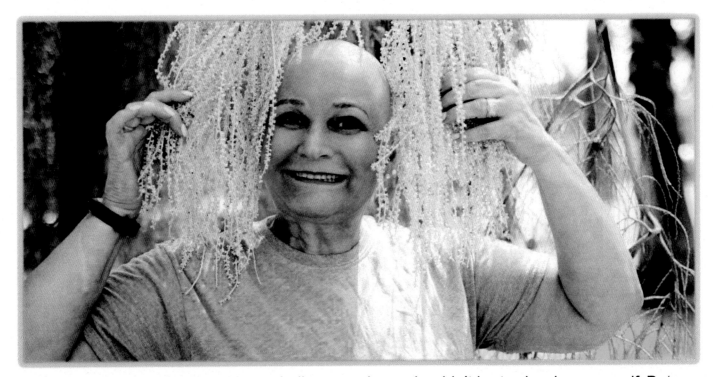

Keeping your spirits up will be a challenge and you shouldn't be too hard on yourself. But sometimes you need to go the extra inch to help yourself achieve a degree of feeling like you've got more going on than just cancer.

If You Don't Have One, Buy a Recliner

While it's important to move your body as much as you can, when you run out of steam (and you will), go to a real brick-and-mortar store and try a few on for size. You'll find shopping for a recliner will feel like you've tumbled right into "Goldilocks and the Three Bears"—some will be too big, some will be too small. Keep going until you find one that is just right.

You're going to be very tired a good part of the time that you're going through chemo, radiation, and their aftermath. You could go back to bed every time you flag, but I found it much better for my sense of "I'm Still Standing" (*à la* Elton John) if, instead of lying down every time I was tired, I merely tilted back my recliner for a snooze. The feeling that you are merely resting instead of collapsing makes you feel less infirm.

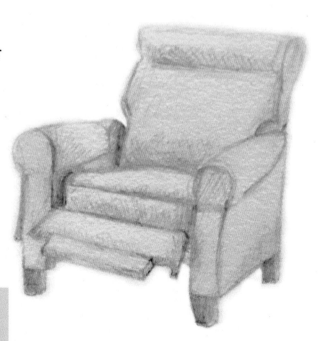

This is absolutely my own advice—no medical professional is going to send you out for a chair.

Exercise Your Mind & Creativity

It's also important to keep your mind occupied with thoughts other than "This Cancer Thing Blows." Staying positive might not be your strong suit through this, so you may find you need a little mental nudge.

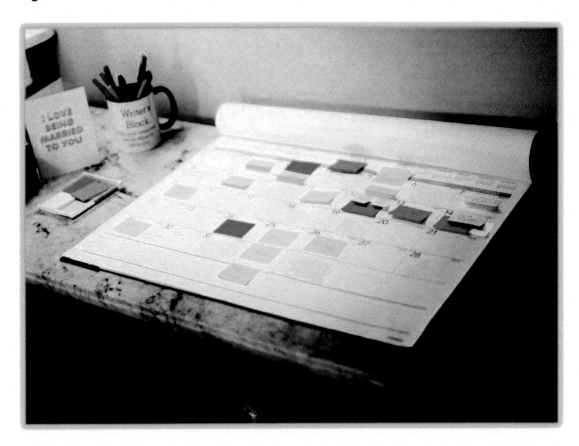

I knew from very early days that I would stumble upon a project I could work on during chemo—or force the issue, if need be.

One day, while I was still at my job on *House Hunters*, I was talking with my boss about a complex shoot I was about to embark upon. He happens to be a bald man. The fact that I had very recently been diagnosed with breast cancer should not have prevented me from keeping my mind on my work, but . . . well, come on! Instead of listening to my boss solve the problem I had come in with, I stared at his bald pate and thought, "This is very interesting. He is bald. He is still handsome. He is still smart. Nobody thinks less of him because he has no hair . . ."

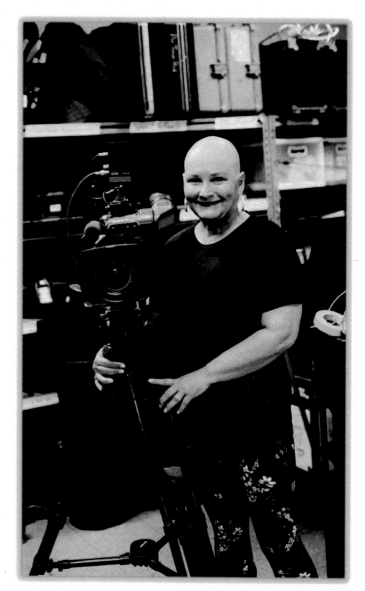

BALD SUPPORT

And with that revelation, my creative project was born. Instead of yet another photo essay on WOMEN WITHOUT HAIR, I would ask all of my bald men-friends, my bald co-workers, and my bald husband to take pictures with me. I also asked them for thoughts about losing their hair. You'd be surprised how many of them didn't just shrug their shoulders as their hair fell out upon those shoulders. Some of them felt just as badly as we do. The fact that society turns a blind eye toward baldness in men didn't always make it easier—and sometimes made it worse.

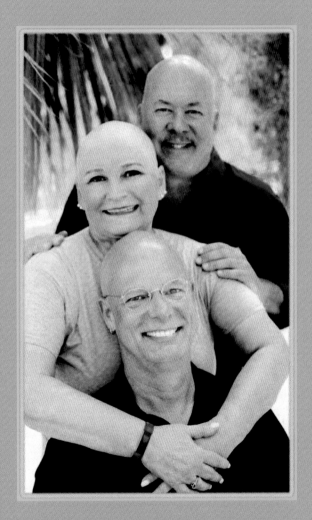

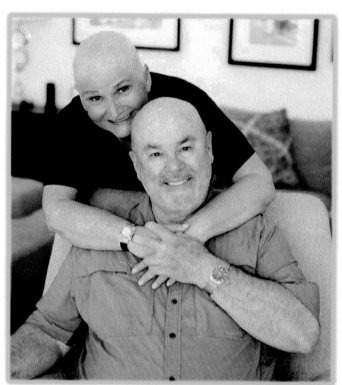
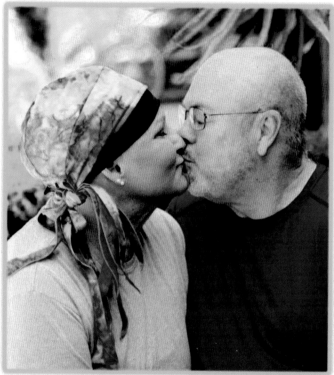

"I knew I was going to be bald because my mother's father was bald.
Science disproved that . . . But by that time, I was bald anyway."
—Billy, Husband

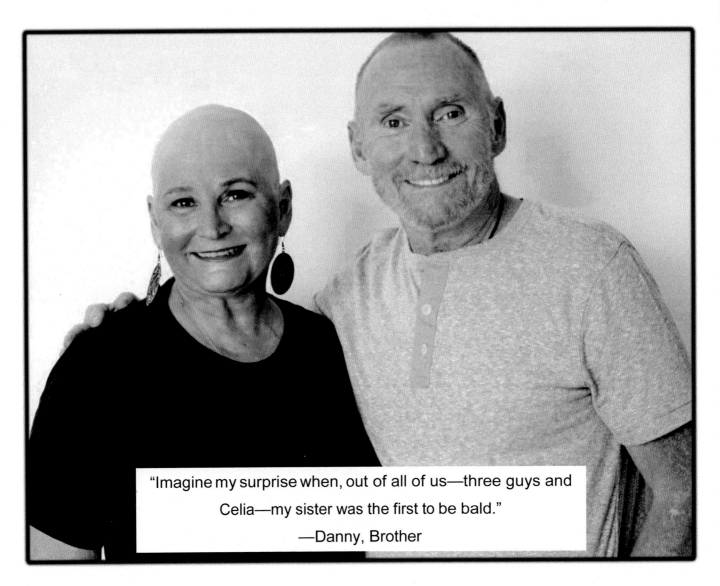

"Imagine my surprise when, out of all of us—three guys and Celia—my sister was the first to be bald."

—Danny, Brother

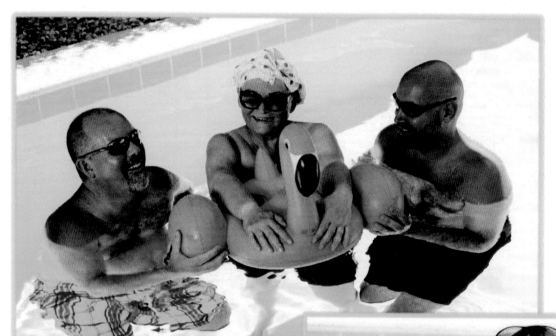

"In the gay community, it's fine to be bald."
—Stephen, Video Producer

"I'm bald?"
—Sean, Financial Advisor

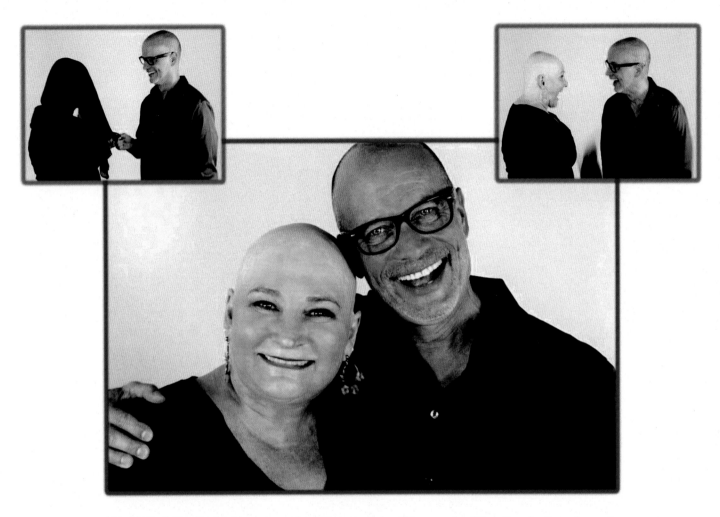

"I think I started to lose my hair in my late 30s, early 40s. I'm lucky since I have a nice shaped noggin. I think it looks kind of sexy and works for me."

—George, TV Colleague

"My attitude about my baldness is 'big deal.'
I lost a generation of friends to AIDS. I have
the privilege of growing old that they didn't.
I'm not going to complain about my hair."
—Michael, Fellow Writer

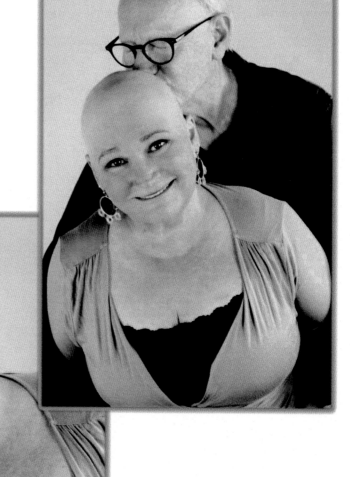

"Because my dad never let me grow my hair, I rebelled when I left home at 18. Little did I know that five years later I'd be losing it."
—Steve, TV Director

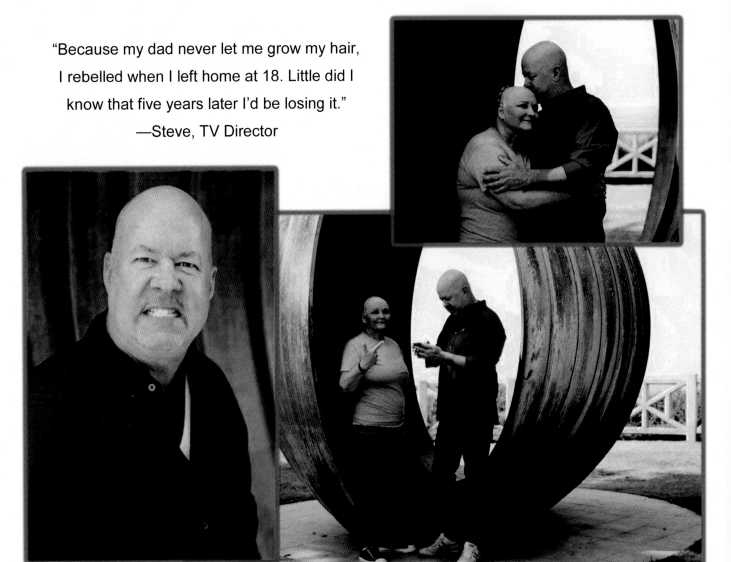

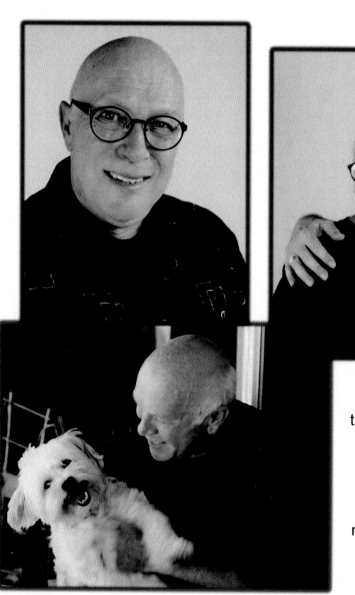

"I was devastated when I went bald! I was trying to get work as an actor. I wore full wigs for years. Consequently, I never let anyone get close. I'm still not crazy about it but it's been this way for over 40 years. Certainly makes getting ready in the morning quicker."

—Jay, Singer

"If hair makes the man,

I'm in trouble."

—Russell, Fiber Artist

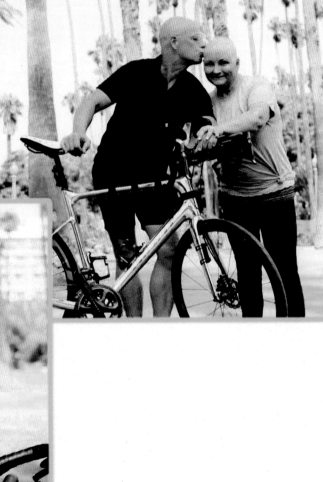

"I spend no money at a hair salon. My 'hair' dries almost instantly. And I have no bad hair days."
—Jeff, TV Colleague

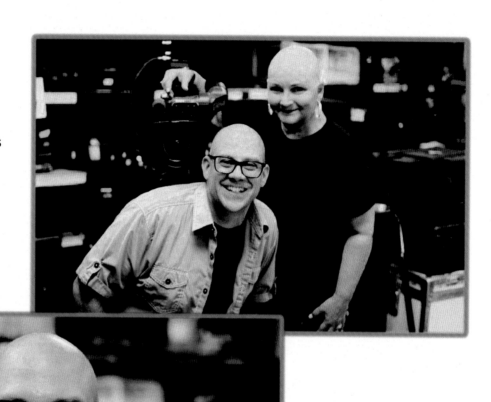

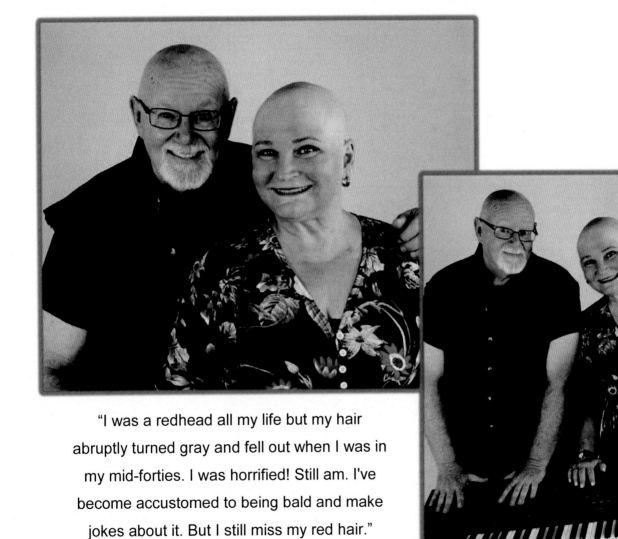

"I was a redhead all my life but my hair abruptly turned gray and fell out when I was in my mid-forties. I was horrified! Still am. I've become accustomed to being bald and make jokes about it. But I still miss my red hair."
—Wayne, Musician

"I shave a lot of women's heads, but this is Los Angeles. Sometimes it's for chemo, but mostly it's for a movie role."
—Victor, Barber

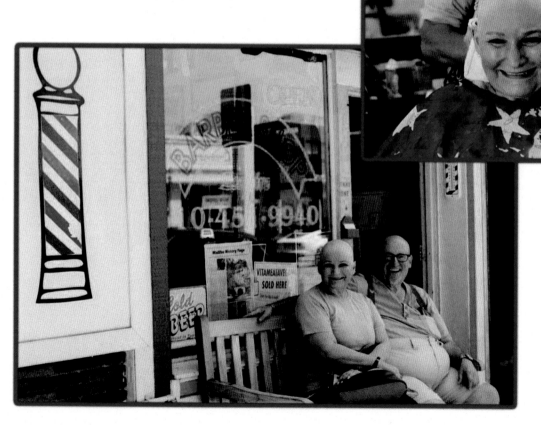

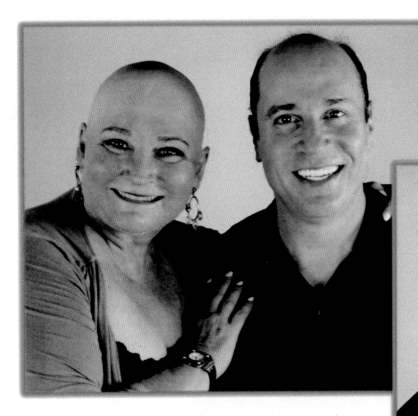

"I let my baldness define weakness and deficiency in my early 20s. I look in the mirror today and do not see a bald man but instead a precious and deserving person."

—Andrew, Therapist

POST-CHEMO

My father once said to me, "When you're a young, naïve dad, you think you're going to worry about your kid for 18 years. But you never stop worrying. It's a lifelong career being a parent."

This holds true for your journey through cancer, as well. When you start, if you are like me, you will be naïve. You will think, "I just need to get through this and everything will return to normal." It will not. It's a lifelong career, being a cancer survivor.

Your hair will likely come back very different from what it was before you went into chemo. Think of this as a metaphor for every part of you. You will have been through the fire. You will come out the other side stronger, more resilient, more patient, less afraid of the world, and less likely to take anything good for granted. You will have a new respect for how precious time is. You've proven your mettle, even if you didn't know that's what you were doing.

Do not mourn the loss of your more innocent self.

Celebrate the warrior you have become.

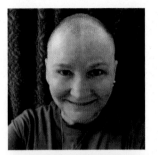
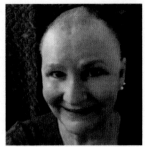
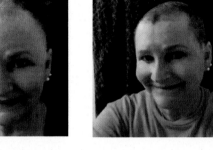
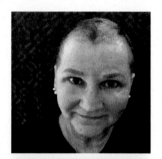

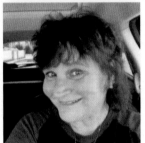
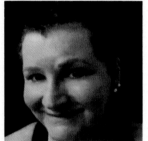

When you are bald, you will promise the Follicle Gods that once you have hair again, you will not complain about whatever they deem fit to send to your head. Chances are good that, if you had thick hair, it will come back thin. If it was straight, it will come back curly. You'll need to remind yourself that the Follicle Gods are not real, because, trust me, you're going to go back on this promise.

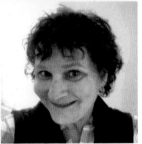
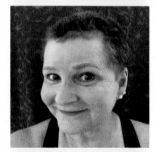

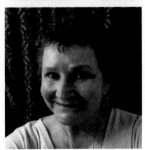
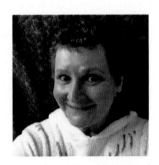
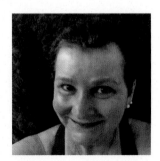
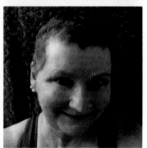

When You No Longer Need Your Scarves, Turbans, or Wigs

The team at Chemocessories believes it is very important to help women feel positive. Their philosophy is that treatment in no way diminishes the beautiful woman within. By putting together sets of scarves, turbans, and jewelry and donating them to women going through treatment, Chemocessories provides women in chemotherapy with a lift to the spirit.

Chemocessories:

www.chemocessories.org

I had a ton of scarves and turbans to give away—and, sadly, I had no shortage of friends who were in need of some beautiful accessories. Should you be fortunate enough to have a completely healthy circle of friends and family, this organization proved to be as awesome as they sound. They'll take your donations and add jewelry and other accessories to create "gift sets" for women in need of a boost.

Cutting Turbans

Once you have a little hair back on your head, you'll be itching to pay it forward with your head coverings. There are many places to donate. I surprised myself by actually wanting to keep a couple of my scarves and turbans. The scarves could live their own lives and, while I never wanted to go back to full-on turban mode, I cut out the top of the turbans and made cute headbands. It was as if my head covering fashions evolved with my health.

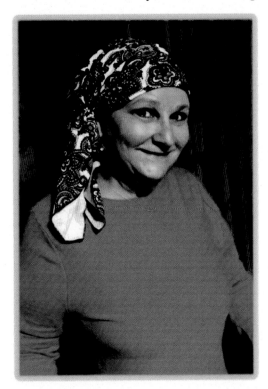 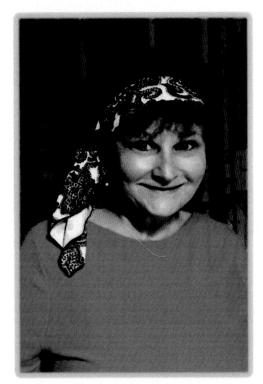

TIPS FROM SOME PINK SISTERS

While I wanted to pass along chemo-easing tips from my own experience, my *pink sisters* also weighed in with some excellent thoughts.

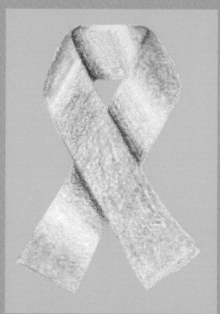

"I bought several different colors of gauze material and taught myself how to wrap my head when I went bald. I also washed and conditioned my scalp with Nioxin. It helped strengthen my hair once it started growing back."

—Linda (Tulsa, OK)

"After a couple months I decided it did not serve me to feel sorry for myself. Best thing I ever did— made the surgery and chemo a whole lot easier."

—Mel (Boynton Beach, FL)

"During chemo, I found satin pillowcases and soft pillows were great for tender skin. A small, fluffy pillow in cool satin can be tucked under your arm, put under your head with no hair, in between your legs. Wherever heat strikes!"

—Cookie (Drummond, CO)

"Fight like a girl for strength and always be kind."

—*Laquita (Coalinga, CA)*

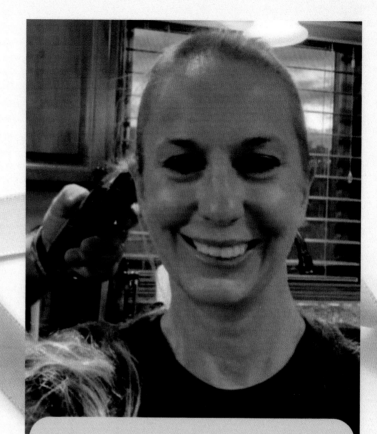

"Several of my friends gave me coloring books. They really made the time go faster. I loved colored pencils and would make sure my points were sharp before every infusion."

—*Belinda (Oklahoma City, OK)*

"Buzzing off hair. Just like everyone says— it feels liberating! I feel strong! Leading up to this was emotional and I wasn't sure how I would feel, but I feel great!"

—*Kristi (Bismarck, ND)*

"Hey, ladies! I wanted to be sure you all know that Target offers an entire line of post-mastectomy swimwear. The adjustable straps some of them offer could be helpful after lumpectomy as well."

—Vanessa (Glendale Heights, IL)

"Get up each day and say 'I can do this.' Remind yourself it's just a bump in the road and you will get through this."

—Cyndy (Bostwick, PA)

"Tell yourself you're beautiful. Don't compare yourself to what you looked liked two months ago because this is your new you. You're going through a transformation that will mold you to a strength only another breast cancer survivor can know."

—Nya (Trenton, NJ)

"If you're alone or living with a non-cook, look into Meal Train, a website set up to help you or one of your helpful friends order meals. It's fast and easy and so very welcome."

—Virginia (Aqua Dulce, CA)

"A friend bought me a nausea pregnancy bracelet called Sea-Band Mama! If, like me, you get motion sickness, these wrist bands are a plus for travel."

—Carol (Naples, FL)

"My stomach was always upset when I finished an infusion. A can of diluted chicken soup always settled it."

—Laurie (Laguna Beach, CA)

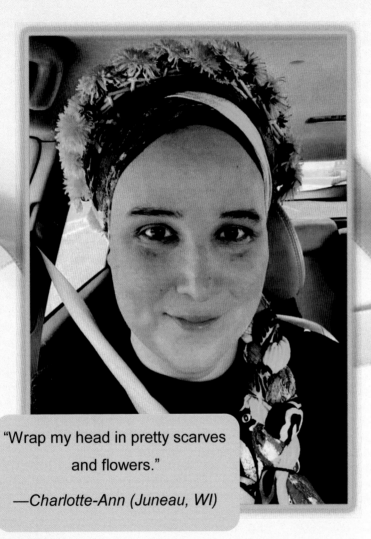

"A sheepskin cover will keep the seatbelt off your port. You can get them online."

—*Lynn (Dallas, TX)*

"Wrap my head in pretty scarves and flowers."

—*Charlotte-Ann (Juneau, WI)*

"I was really happy I included a back scratcher in my chemo bag."

—*Patti (Woodland Hills, CA)*

"I know staying hydrated is key in life—but double so during chemo. For some reason, I couldn't stand plain water, so I drank lightly flavored carbonated water."

—Charlotte (Albany, NY)

"I always seemed to be overheated. I found just one light blanket and a well-made bed helped me to sleep. Sometimes had to leave my husband and settle myself on another comfortable bed when I was too hot and needed to sneak my head piece off."

—Diane (Los Angeles, CA)

"Bring a weighted blanket to chemo. It's comforting and warm."

—Krista (Lexington, MI)

"When I went through chemo, aromas of foods I loved suddenly made me feel queasy. I ate a lot of plain (odorless) oatmeal. Once you introduce maple or cinnamon—forget it."

—Tina (Seattle, WA)

"My taste buds changed continually, but the taste of lemon-lime soda remained a flavor I could always count on."

—Roxanne (Rochester, NY)

"Drink hot tea with sugar or substitutes to get your pills to go down."

—Ann (New York, NY)

"Don't forget: a passport lasts 10 years! If your passport is going to expire in the next year or so, you might want to consider having your photo taken before your hair falls out. There's enough stress getting a decent passport picture without adding how your photograph is going to look for the next decade."

—Louise (Thousand Oaks, CA)

"Post-chemo, I am loving only the taste of tomato ketchup . . . having it with everything, like a toddler."

—Ahlam (New Delhi, India)

A FINAL WORD ABOUT ALL THIS...

During treatment, you will long for the day when you will return to your old self. But this journey is a one-way street. You will not return to the person you were. You are now a warrior. Take your newfound strength and run with it. Do NOT let cancer define you.

Do NOT feel you need to share details of your now-in-remission cancer adventure with someone going through their own current trial, unless it is to offer advice or encouragement.

Above all, listen. This is their time, their story.

Be grateful it is no longer yours.

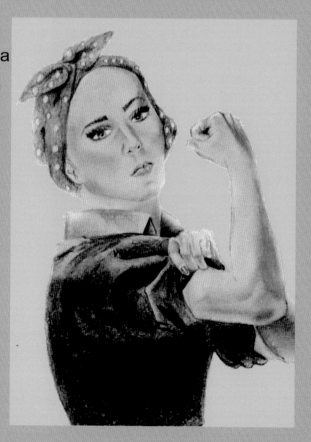

ABOUT THE AUTHOR

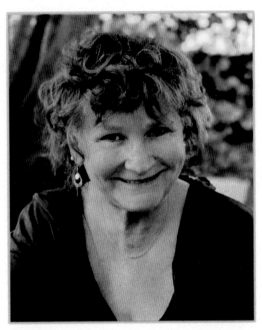

Celia Bonaduce is an award-winning novelist, podcast writer, and television producer. Celia spent fifteen years as a producer-director in lifestyle programming. Her shows include ABC's *Extreme Makeover: Home Edition* and HGTV's *House Hunters* and *Tiny House Hunters*.

As a novelist with Kensington Publishing, Celia has written three trilogies: the Venice Beach Romances, the Fat Chance, Texas series, and the Tiny House Novels. The Tiny House Novel series won top honors with a Grand Finalist nod from the New Apple Official Selection, first place in the Book Excellence Awards, and Gold from both the National Federation of Press Women and the Elite Choice Awards.

Celia is also a co-author of *A Texas Kind of Christmas*, released by Kensington. *A Texas Kind of Christmas* was an Amazon Number 1 Best Seller in Historical Romance and took Gold from the National Federation of Press Women.

Cancer got in the way of traveling for *House Hunters* but did not stop Celia's creativity. While the road to her first nonfiction book was anything but SMOOTH, it was a path that Celia felt compelled to explore.

www.celiabonaduce.com